NUTRITIONAL GUIDELINES FOR MAINTAINING KIDNEY HEALTH

EKELE SUNDAY

ISBN: 9798328618489

DEDICATION

This book is dedicated to my beloved mother, Elizabeth Isaac. You have been the guiding light and unwavering support throughout my life. Your boundless love, wisdom, and strength have shaped not only who I am but also this book. Your encouragement to pursue my dreams has always been a source of inspiration. This book is a tribute to your endless sacrifices and the profound impact you've had on my journey. Thank you for always believing in me.

CONTENTS

Overview of Kidney Health

The kidneys are vital organs that play a crucial role in maintaining our overall health. Located just below the rib cage on either side of the spine, these bean-shaped organs are responsible for filtering waste products and excess fluids from the blood, which are then excreted as urine. In addition to their filtration function, the kidneys help regulate blood pressure, balance electrolytes, produce hormones that influence red blood cell production, and maintain strong bones. Given their critical functions, maintaining kidney health is essential for the body's overall well-being.

Importance of Kidneys in the Human Body

Kidneys are often referred to as the body's natural filtration system. Every day, they filter about 150 quarts of blood to remove about 1 to 2 quarts of waste and extra fluid. This waste includes byproducts from normal metabolic processes, toxins, and excess substances like sodium and potassium. The kidneys also help maintain the body's fluid balance, ensuring that we have the right amount of water and electrolytes to support bodily functions. They release hormones like erythropoietin, which stimulates red blood cell production, and renin, which regulates blood pressure. The kidneys' multifaceted role underscores their importance in sustaining life and health.

How Diet Impacts Kidney Function

Diet plays a pivotal role in maintaining kidney health. What we eat can directly affect how well our kidneys function. Consuming a balanced diet rich in essential nutrients supports the kidneys in filtering blood, maintaining electrolyte balance, and managing waste efficiently. Conversely, a diet high in sodium, phosphorus, and potassium can overburden the kidneys, particularly if they are already compromised by conditions like chronic kidney disease (CKD) or diabetes. Proper hydration, the right amount of protein, and the avoidance of harmful substances are key components of a diet that promotes optimal kidney health.

Purpose of the Book

The purpose of this book, "Nutritional Guidelines for Maintaining Kidney Health," is to provide comprehensive, evidence-based dietary guidance to support kidney function and prevent kidney-related diseases. Whether you are someone looking to maintain healthy kidneys, a patient managing a kidney condition, a caregiver, or a healthcare professional, this book aims to offer valuable insights and practical advice.

Providing Nutritional Guidelines for Kidney Health

This book outlines nutritional guidelines that are specifically designed to support kidney health. It delves into the essential nutrients required by the kidneys, how to balance these nutrients in your diet, and the impact of various foods on kidney function. Each chapter provides detailed information on managing protein, potassium, phosphorus, sodium, and fluid intake, which are critical for individuals with kidney concerns. Additionally, we offer meal planning tips, recipes, and advice on navigating social situations and dining out while adhering to a kidney-friendly diet.

Target Audience: Individuals, Caregivers, Healthcare Professionals

"Nutritional Guidelines for Maintaining Kidney Health" is crafted for a diverse audience. It serves as a practical guide for individuals who aim to maintain their kidney health through diet and for those managing existing kidney conditions. Caregivers will find useful information on how to support their loved ones with dietary adjustments. Healthcare professionals, including dietitians and nurses, can use this book as a resource to assist their patients in making informed dietary choices. By bridging the gap between scientific research and everyday practice, this book empowers readers with the knowledge to take proactive steps in preserving kidney health.

In the chapters that follow, we will explore in detail how the kidneys function, the impact of various nutrients, and practical strategies for incorporating kidney-friendly foods into your daily routine. Whether you are new to the concept of kidney health or looking to deepen your understanding, this book provides the tools you need to nurture your kidneys through mindful nutrition.

UNDERSTANDING THE KIDNEYS

To maintain kidney health through nutrition, it is essential first to understand the anatomy, physiology, and function of the kidneys, as well as common kidney diseases and the impact of diet on these conditions. This chapter provides a comprehensive overview of these topics.

Anatomy and Physiology of the Kidneys

The kidneys are two bean-shaped organs located on either side of the spine, just below the ribcage. They are about the size of a fist and play a critical role in maintaining overall health.

Structure and Function:

- **Nephrons**: Each kidney contains approximately one million nephrons, which are the functional units of the kidney. Nephrons filter blood to produce urine.
- **Renal Cortex and Medulla**: The outer part of the kidney is called the renal cortex, and the inner part is the renal medulla. These areas house the nephrons and collecting ducts.
- **Renal Pelvis**: The central part of the kidney, known as the renal pelvis, collects urine before it flows into the ureter and then to the bladder.

Role in the Body's Waste Management:

- **Filtration**: Blood enters the kidneys through the renal arteries, and waste products, excess substances, and toxins are filtered out through the nephrons.
- **Reabsorption**: Useful substances like glucose, amino acids, and electrolytes are reabsorbed back into the bloodstream.
- **Excretion**: The remaining waste products are excreted as urine, which flows from the kidneys to the bladder via the ureters and is eventually expelled from the body.

Common Kidney Diseases

Kidneys are susceptible to various diseases, which can significantly impact their function and overall health. Understanding these diseases is crucial for effective dietary management.

Chronic Kidney Disease (CKD):

- **Overview**: CKD is a gradual loss of kidney function over time. It can progress to end-stage renal disease (ESRD), requiring dialysis or a kidney transplant.
- **Causes**: Diabetes and hypertension are the leading causes of CKD. Other causes include glomerulonephritis, polycystic kidney disease, and prolonged obstruction of the urinary tract.
- **Symptoms**: Early stages may have no symptoms. As the disease progresses, symptoms include fatigue, swelling, changes in urine output, and high blood pressure.

Kidney Stones:

- **Overview**: Kidney stones are hard deposits of minerals and salts that form in the kidneys. They can cause severe pain and urinary issues.
- **Types**: The most common types are calcium oxalate stones, uric acid stones, struvite stones, and cystine stones.
- **Causes**: Factors include dehydration, certain diets (high in protein, salt, or sugar), obesity, and specific medical conditions.
- **Symptoms**: Symptoms include severe pain in the side and back, blood in urine, nausea, and frequent urination.

How Diet Influences These Conditions

Diet plays a vital role in both the prevention and management of kidney diseases. Understanding the impact of different nutrients and dietary patterns can help maintain kidney health and prevent complications.

Chronic Kidney Disease (CKD):

- **Protein**: Excessive protein intake can strain the kidneys. A moderate protein diet, often guided by a healthcare provider, is recommended for individuals with CKD.

- **Sodium**: High sodium intake can increase blood pressure and worsen kidney damage. A low-sodium diet helps manage blood pressure and fluid balance.
- **Potassium and Phosphorus**: CKD patients may need to limit potassium and phosphorus intake to prevent complications like hyperkalemia and hyperphosphatemia.
- **Hydration**: Proper hydration is essential to help the kidneys function efficiently but must be balanced to avoid fluid overload.

Kidney Stones:

- **Calcium**: Contrary to popular belief, a low-calcium diet can increase the risk of kidney stones. A diet with adequate calcium can help prevent stone formation.
- **Oxalates**: Foods high in oxalates, such as spinach, nuts, and tea, should be limited for individuals prone to calcium oxalate stones.
- **Protein**: High animal protein intake can increase the risk of stone formation. A diet with moderate protein from plant sources is often recommended.
- **Hydration**: Drinking plenty of water dilutes substances in the urine that lead to stones. Aim for at least 2-3 liters of water per day.

By understanding the structure, function, and diseases of the kidneys, along with the significant impact of diet on kidney health, you can make informed dietary choices to support and maintain kidney function. The following chapters will delve deeper into specific nutrients and dietary strategies to optimize kidney health.

Basics of Kidney-Friendly Nutrition

Proper nutrition is fundamental to maintaining healthy kidneys and preventing or managing kidney disease. Understanding which nutrients are essential and how to balance them in your diet is crucial for supporting kidney function. In this chapter, we will explore the essential nutrients for kidney health, the specific roles of protein, potassium, phosphorus, sodium, and fluids, and provide practical dietary recommendations. Balancing these nutrients effectively and ensuring adequate hydration are key steps toward maintaining optimal kidney health.

1. Essential Nutrients for Kidney Health

Kidneys require a variety of nutrients to function efficiently and sustain overall health. These essential nutrients include:

- **Protein**: Vital for tissue repair and maintenance, but needs to be carefully managed to avoid overburdening the kidneys.
- **Potassium**: Important for nerve and muscle function, but must be balanced to prevent hyperkalemia or hypokalemia.
- **Phosphorus**: Necessary for bone health and energy production, but excess phosphorus can lead to bone and cardiovascular problems in kidney patients.
- **Sodium**: Crucial for fluid balance and nerve function, but excessive intake can lead to hypertension and fluid retention.
- **Fluids**: Essential for waste removal and maintaining blood volume, but fluid intake must be tailored to individual needs, especially in those with kidney disease.

Understanding how each of these nutrients affects kidney function helps in creating a diet that supports kidney health without causing additional strain.

2. Protein, Potassium, Phosphorus, Sodium, and Fluids

Each of these nutrients plays a significant role in kidney health, and managing their intake is vital for both prevention and treatment of kidney-related issues.

Protein:

- **Role**: Protein is necessary for growth, repair, and maintenance of body tissues. It also supports immune function and hormone production.
- **Management**: Excessive protein intake can increase the kidneys' workload. People with kidney disease often need to limit their protein intake to prevent further damage.

Potassium:

- **Role**: Potassium helps regulate heart and muscle function, and maintains fluid and electrolyte balance.
- **Management**: High potassium levels can be dangerous for people with kidney disease, as their kidneys may not effectively remove excess potassium, leading to hyperkalemia.

Phosphorus:

- **Role**: Phosphorus is essential for bone health and energy production.
- **Management**: In kidney disease, phosphorus can accumulate in the blood, leading to bone and heart problems. It's important to monitor and limit phosphorus intake.

Sodium:

- **Role**: Sodium controls fluid balance, nerve impulses, and muscle function.
- **Management**: High sodium intake can cause high blood pressure and fluid retention, straining the kidneys. Reducing sodium intake helps manage these risks.

Fluids:

- **Role**: Fluids help the kidneys filter waste from the blood and maintain overall fluid balance.
- **Management**: Adequate hydration is important, but in kidney disease, fluid intake may need to be restricted to prevent fluid overload.

3. Dietary Recommendations for Kidney Health

Following dietary recommendations tailored for kidney health can help maintain kidney function and prevent further complications. Key recommendations include:

- **Protein**: Choose high-quality protein sources such as lean meats, fish, eggs, and plant-based proteins. Adjust protein intake based on kidney function and medical advice.
- **Potassium**: Focus on low-potassium fruits and vegetables such as apples, berries, carrots, and green beans. Avoid high-potassium foods like bananas, oranges, potatoes, and tomatoes if advised.
- **Phosphorus**: Limit foods high in phosphorus like dairy products, nuts, seeds, and colas. Opt for phosphorus binders if prescribed by a healthcare provider.
- **Sodium**: Use herbs and spices instead of salt to flavor food. Avoid processed and packaged foods, which are often high in sodium.
- **Fluids**: Drink adequate amounts of water, but follow your healthcare provider's advice on fluid restrictions if you have kidney disease.

4. Balancing Nutrients

Balancing nutrients involves ensuring you get the right amounts of each essential nutrient without overloading the kidneys. This requires:

- **Planning Meals**: Create a balanced meal plan that includes a variety of nutrient-dense foods while controlling portions of protein, potassium, phosphorus, and sodium.
- **Reading Labels**: Learn to read food labels to track nutrient intake, particularly sodium, phosphorus, and potassium.
- **Working with a Dietitian**: Consult a renal dietitian who can tailor dietary recommendations to your specific needs and kidney function.

Balancing nutrients helps in maintaining kidney health and preventing complications from improper nutrient intake.

5. Importance of Hydration

Hydration plays a crucial role in kidney health by aiding in the removal of waste products and maintaining overall fluid balance. Here's why hydration is important and how to manage it:

- **Waste Removal**: Proper hydration ensures that the kidneys can efficiently filter and remove waste products from the blood.
- **Preventing Kidney Stones**: Adequate fluid intake helps prevent the formation of kidney stones by diluting the urine.
- **Managing Fluid Balance**: In kidney disease, managing fluid intake is vital to avoid fluid overload and related complications.

Tips for Staying Hydrated:

- Drink water throughout the day rather than large amounts at once.
- Monitor fluid intake if you have been advised to restrict fluids.
- Avoid sugary drinks and limit caffeine and alcohol, which can dehydrate the body.

In conclusion, understanding the basics of kidney-friendly nutrition and implementing these dietary guidelines can significantly impact kidney health. By focusing on essential nutrients, managing protein, potassium, phosphorus, sodium, and fluids, and ensuring proper hydration, you can support your kidneys in performing their vital functions effectively.

THE ROLE OF PROTEIN

Protein is a vital nutrient that plays numerous roles in maintaining overall health, including supporting muscle and tissue repair, immune function, and hormone production. For individuals concerned about kidney health, understanding protein needs and managing protein intake is crucial. In this chapter, we will explore the importance of protein for kidney health, recommended daily intake, sources of kidney-friendly proteins, the differences between plant-based and animal-based proteins, and the best sources and portion sizes for a kidney-friendly diet.

1. Understanding Protein Needs

Protein is composed of amino acids, which are the building blocks of the body's cells and tissues. It is essential for growth, repair, and maintaining bodily functions. However, the body's requirement for protein varies based on several factors, including age, sex, physical activity level, and health status.

For individuals with kidney concerns, protein needs can be different. Healthy kidneys efficiently filter and excrete the byproducts of protein metabolism. In people with impaired kidney function, excessive protein intake can increase the workload on the kidneys, potentially accelerating the progression of kidney disease. Therefore, understanding and managing protein needs is key to maintaining kidney health.

2. Importance for Kidney Health

While protein is necessary for overall health, its impact on kidney function requires careful consideration. Here's why protein is important for kidney health:

- **Repair and Maintenance**: Protein helps repair and maintain tissues, including those in the kidneys. Adequate protein intake supports recovery and maintenance of kidney function.

- **Immune Support**: Protein plays a critical role in the immune system, helping to fight infections that could potentially harm the kidneys.
- **Hormone Production**: Proteins are involved in producing hormones and enzymes that regulate various bodily functions, including those related to kidney function.

However, for individuals with chronic kidney disease (CKD), managing protein intake is essential to reduce the burden on the kidneys and slow disease progression.

3. Recommended Daily Intake

The recommended daily intake of protein varies based on individual health status and kidney function. General guidelines for protein intake are as follows:

- **Healthy Adults**: The Recommended Dietary Allowance (RDA) for protein is about 0.8 grams per kilogram of body weight. For example, a person weighing 70 kg (154 lbs) would need about 56 grams of protein per day.
- **Chronic Kidney Disease (CKD)**: Protein intake may need to be reduced to 0.6-0.8 grams per kilogram of body weight per day, depending on the stage of CKD and medical advice.
- **Dialysis Patients**: Individuals on dialysis may require higher protein intake, about 1.2-1.4 grams per kilogram of body weight per day, to compensate for protein loss during dialysis treatments.

It is essential to consult with a healthcare provider or renal dietitian to determine the appropriate protein intake based on individual needs and kidney function.

4. Sources of Kidney-Friendly Proteins

Choosing the right sources of protein is crucial for maintaining kidney health. Kidney-friendly proteins are those that provide high-quality amino acids while minimizing the burden on the kidneys. These sources include:

- **Lean Meats**: Chicken, turkey, and lean cuts of beef or pork.
- **Fish**: Salmon, tuna, and other low-mercury fish.
- **Eggs**: Whole eggs and egg whites.

- **Dairy**: Low-phosphorus options like Greek yogurt and cottage cheese.

In addition to these animal-based sources, plant-based proteins are also beneficial and often lower in phosphorus and potassium, making them suitable for kidney health.

5. Plant-Based vs. Animal-Based Proteins

Both plant-based and animal-based proteins have their benefits and considerations for kidney health.

Plant-Based Proteins:

- **Benefits**: Often lower in phosphorus and potassium, high in fiber, and contain beneficial antioxidants.
- **Sources**: Beans, lentils, tofu, tempeh, quinoa, nuts, and seeds.
- **Considerations**: Some plant-based proteins are high in potassium and phosphorus, so portion control and proper preparation (e.g., soaking beans) are important.

Animal-Based Proteins:

- **Benefits**: Provide complete proteins with all essential amino acids, easily absorbed by the body.
- **Sources**: Lean meats, fish, eggs, and dairy products.
- **Considerations**: Often higher in phosphorus and cholesterol, so choosing lean and low-fat options is recommended.

Balancing plant-based and animal-based proteins can provide a variety of nutrients while supporting kidney health.

6. Best Sources and Portion Sizes

Selecting the best sources of protein and managing portion sizes is crucial for a kidney-friendly diet. Here are some of the best sources and appropriate portion sizes:

- **Chicken Breast**: 3 ounces (about the size of a deck of cards) provides approximately 21 grams of protein.

- **Fish (e.g., Salmon)**: 3 ounces provides about 22 grams of protein.
- **Eggs**: One large egg provides about 6 grams of protein.
- **Greek Yogurt**: 1 cup provides about 10 grams of protein.
- **Tofu**: ½ cup provides about 10 grams of protein.
- **Lentils**: ½ cup cooked provides about 9 grams of protein.
- **Quinoa**: 1 cup cooked provides about 8 grams of protein.

Portion sizes should be adjusted based on individual protein needs and kidney function. It's important to balance protein intake with other nutrients to ensure a well-rounded diet.

In conclusion, understanding the role of protein in kidney health, managing protein intake, and selecting the right sources are crucial steps in maintaining optimal kidney function. By focusing on kidney-friendly proteins, balancing plant-based and animal-based sources, and adhering to recommended portion sizes, individuals can support their kidneys while enjoying a nutritious and varied diet.

Managing Potassium and Phosphorus Intake

Maintaining the right balance of potassium and phosphorus is essential for kidney health. These minerals are vital for various bodily functions, but imbalances can cause significant health issues, particularly for individuals with kidney disease. In this chapter, we will explore the dual nature of potassium and phosphorus, their importance for body function, and strategies for managing their levels to support kidney health.

1. Potassium: Friend and Foe

Potassium is a critical mineral that plays a key role in maintaining normal cell function, particularly in the heart, muscles, and nerves. However, when kidney function is impaired, managing potassium levels becomes crucial. Too much or too little potassium can have severe health implications, making it both a friend and a foe.

2. Importance for Body Function

Potassium is essential for several bodily functions, including:

- **Nerve Function**: It helps transmit nerve impulses, which are necessary for muscle contractions and other bodily functions.
- **Muscle Contraction**: Potassium is crucial for muscle function, including the muscles of the heart, which relies on proper potassium levels to maintain a regular heartbeat.
- **Fluid Balance**: It helps maintain the balance of fluids in the body's cells and tissues.
- **Blood Pressure Regulation**: Potassium works with sodium to regulate blood pressure. Adequate potassium can help counteract the effects of sodium and reduce blood pressure.

Given its importance, maintaining the right level of potassium is vital for overall health and well-being.

3. Managing High and Low Potassium Levels

Managing potassium levels is particularly important for individuals with kidney disease, as their kidneys may struggle to maintain appropriate potassium levels.

High Potassium Levels (Hyperkalemia):

- **Causes**: Reduced kidney function, high potassium intake, certain medications.
- **Symptoms**: Muscle weakness, fatigue, irregular heartbeat, and in severe cases, cardiac arrest.
- **Management**:
    - **Dietary Adjustments**: Limit high-potassium foods such as bananas, oranges, potatoes, tomatoes, and spinach.
    - **Medication**: Potassium binders may be prescribed to help reduce potassium levels.
    - **Dialysis**: In severe cases, dialysis may be required to remove excess potassium from the blood.

Low Potassium Levels (Hypokalemia):

- **Causes**: Inadequate dietary intake, excessive loss due to vomiting or diarrhea, certain medications.
- **Symptoms**: Muscle cramps, weakness, fatigue, irregular heartbeats.
- **Management**:
    - **Dietary Adjustments**: Increase intake of potassium-rich foods such as bananas, oranges, and potatoes if not contraindicated by kidney function.
    - **Supplements**: Potassium supplements may be prescribed under medical supervision.

Balancing potassium intake requires careful monitoring and adjustments based on individual health conditions and medical advice.

4. Phosphorus: Balancing Act

Phosphorus is another essential mineral that plays a crucial role in the body but must be carefully managed, especially for those with kidney disease. An imbalance in phosphorus levels can lead to significant health issues, making its management a delicate balancing act.

5. Role in the Body

Phosphorus is vital for several key functions, including:

- **Bone Health**: It works with calcium to build and maintain strong bones and teeth.
- **Energy Production**: Phosphorus is a component of ATP (adenosine triphosphate), which provides energy for cellular processes.
- **Cell Structure**: It is a part of DNA, RNA, and cell membranes, essential for cellular function and replication.
- **Acid-Base Balance**: Phosphorus helps maintain the body's acid-base balance.

Given its critical roles, maintaining appropriate phosphorus levels is essential for overall health.

6. Avoiding High-Phosphorus Foods

For individuals with kidney disease, managing phosphorus intake is crucial to prevent complications such as bone disease and cardiovascular problems. Here are strategies to avoid high-phosphorus foods:

High-Phosphorus Foods to Avoid:

- **Dairy Products**: Milk, cheese, yogurt, and other dairy products are high in phosphorus.
- **Processed Foods**: Many processed and packaged foods contain added phosphorus as preservatives.
- **Meats and Fish**: Organ meats and certain fish like sardines and salmon contain high levels of phosphorus.
- **Nuts and Seeds**: Almonds, sunflower seeds, and other nuts and seeds are high in phosphorus.
- **Beans and Lentils**: These are healthy but can be high in phosphorus and should be consumed in moderation.

Tips for Managing Phosphorus Intake:

- **Read Labels**: Check food labels for phosphorus additives, which often appear as ingredients ending in "-phosphate."

- **Choose Fresh Foods**: Fresh, unprocessed foods generally contain lower levels of phosphorus compared to processed foods.
- **Limit Dairy**: Opt for low-phosphorus alternatives like almond milk, rice milk, or other non-dairy options.
- **Cook from Scratch**: Preparing meals at home allows better control over ingredients and phosphorus content.

Phosphate Binders: For individuals with chronic kidney disease, phosphate binders may be prescribed. These medications help bind phosphorus in the digestive tract, reducing its absorption and helping to maintain lower phosphorus levels in the blood.

In conclusion, managing potassium and phosphorus intake is vital for maintaining kidney health. Understanding the roles of these minerals, recognizing the signs of imbalances, and making dietary adjustments can significantly impact kidney function and overall well-being. By avoiding high-potassium and high-phosphorus foods, and following medical advice, individuals can effectively manage their nutrient intake to support their kidney health.

Sodium and Fluid Management

Managing sodium intake and maintaining proper fluid balance are crucial components of a kidney-friendly diet. Both sodium and fluids play significant roles in kidney health, particularly in managing blood pressure and supporting overall kidney function. In this chapter, we will explore the impact of sodium on kidney health, its role in blood pressure regulation, tips for reducing sodium intake, fluid management strategies, the importance of proper hydration, and recommended fluid intake and sources for optimal kidney health.

1. Impact of Sodium on Kidney Health

Sodium is an essential mineral that helps maintain fluid balance in the body. However, excessive sodium intake can lead to high blood pressure (hypertension) and fluid retention, both of which can strain the kidneys over time. For individuals with kidney disease, reducing sodium intake is crucial to help manage blood pressure and reduce the risk of fluid overload.

2. Sodium's Role in Blood Pressure Regulation

Sodium plays a significant role in regulating blood pressure. When sodium levels are high, the body retains water to dilute the sodium concentration in the bloodstream. This excess fluid increases blood volume and puts strain on blood vessels and the heart, leading to elevated blood pressure. High blood pressure is a risk factor for kidney disease progression and cardiovascular complications.

3. Tips for Reducing Sodium Intake

Reducing sodium intake can help manage blood pressure and support kidney health. Here are some tips to lower sodium intake:

- **Read Food Labels**: Choose low-sodium or sodium-free options when available. Pay attention to serving sizes and sodium content per serving.

- **Cook at Home**: Prepare meals from scratch using fresh ingredients to control sodium levels. Limit the use of salt and high-sodium condiments.
- **Limit Processed Foods**: Processed and packaged foods often contain high levels of sodium. Choose fresh fruits and vegetables, lean meats, and low-sodium alternatives.
- **Use Herbs and Spices**: Flavor foods with herbs, spices, lemon juice, or vinegar instead of salt.
- **Avoid Salt at the Table**: Limit adding salt to meals during cooking or at the table.
- **Choose Low-Sodium Products**: Opt for low-sodium or sodium-free versions of canned soups, sauces, and snacks.

By reducing sodium intake, individuals can help manage blood pressure and lessen the strain on their kidneys.

4. Fluid Management

Proper fluid management is essential for kidney health, especially for individuals with kidney disease. The kidneys regulate fluid balance by adjusting urine production based on the body's needs. Fluid management strategies include:

- **Monitor Fluid Intake**: Keep track of daily fluid intake, including beverages and foods with high water content.
- **Follow Medical Recommendations**: Individuals with kidney disease may need to restrict fluids to prevent fluid overload and complications like edema and high blood pressure.
- **Balance Hydration**: Drink fluids throughout the day rather than large amounts at once. Adjust fluid intake based on activity level, climate, and medical advice.
- **Limit Fluids in the Evening**: Reduce fluid intake in the evening to prevent nighttime bathroom trips that may disrupt sleep.

5. Importance of Proper Hydration

Proper hydration is crucial for kidney health as it supports the kidneys in filtering waste products from the blood and maintaining overall fluid balance. Adequate hydration helps prevent kidney stones by diluting urine and reducing the concentration of minerals that can crystallize and form stones.

6. Recommended Fluid Intake and Sources

The recommended fluid intake varies based on individual factors such as age, sex, climate, and activity level. General guidelines for fluid intake to support kidney health include:

- **Water**: Drink plain water as the primary source of fluids. Aim for at least 8-10 cups (about 2-2.5 liters) of fluids per day, adjusting based on individual needs and medical advice.
- **Herbal Teas**: Unsweetened herbal teas can contribute to fluid intake without added sugars or caffeine.
- **Fruits and Vegetables**: Many fruits and vegetables have high water content and can contribute to daily fluid intake. Examples include cucumbers, watermelon, oranges, and celery.
- **Limit Caffeine and Alcohol**: Caffeine and alcohol can have diuretic effects, increasing urine production and potentially affecting fluid balance. Limit intake as advised by healthcare providers.

By maintaining proper hydration and managing sodium intake, individuals can support kidney function and overall health. Following these guidelines helps reduce the risk of complications associated with kidney disease and promotes overall well-being.

VITAMINS AND MINERALS

Vitamins and minerals are crucial for maintaining kidney health and overall well-being. This chapter delves into the essential micronutrients necessary for supporting kidney function, their specific roles in the body, and sources with recommended intake levels to guide individuals in maintaining optimal nutrition for kidney health.

1. Essential Micronutrients for Kidney Health

Micronutrients, such as vitamins and minerals, are vital for various physiological processes that impact kidney health. Key micronutrients essential for kidney health include:

- **Vitamin D**: Essential for calcium absorption and bone health. Adequate vitamin D levels are crucial for preventing bone disorders like renal osteodystrophy.
- **Vitamin B Complex (B1, B2, B6, B12)**: Important for energy metabolism, nerve function, and red blood cell production, supporting overall vitality and reducing fatigue.
- **Vitamin C**: Acts as an antioxidant, protecting cells from damage caused by free radicals and supporting immune function.
- **Folate (Vitamin B9)**: Essential for DNA synthesis and cell division, promoting overall cellular health and repair.
- **Calcium**: Critical for maintaining bone strength and muscle function. It plays a role in nerve transmission and blood clotting.
- **Magnesium**: Supports muscle and nerve function, regulates blood sugar levels, and aids in energy production.
- **Iron**: Vital for oxygen transport in the blood and essential for the formation of hemoglobin in red blood cells.
- **Zinc**: Supports immune function, wound healing, and cell division, contributing to overall immune health and vitality.

These micronutrients play diverse and vital roles in maintaining overall health, particularly in individuals with compromised kidney function who may have specific dietary needs.

2. Role of Specific Vitamins and Minerals

Each vitamin and mineral contributes uniquely to kidney health and overall bodily functions:

- **Vitamin D**: Regulates calcium and phosphorus metabolism, crucial for bone health and preventing mineral imbalances that can impact kidney function.
- **Vitamin B Complex**: Supports energy metabolism, nerve function, and the production of red blood cells, aiding in the prevention of anemia and promoting overall vitality.
- **Vitamin C**: Acts as an antioxidant, protecting cells from oxidative stress and supporting immune function to help combat infections.
- **Folate**: Essential for DNA synthesis and cell division, critical for growth, repair, and overall cellular health.
- **Calcium**: Maintains bone strength and density, supports muscle function, and plays a role in hormone secretion and nerve transmission.
- **Magnesium**: Supports muscle and nerve function, regulates blood sugar levels, and contributes to energy production and protein synthesis.
- **Iron**: Facilitates oxygen transport in the blood, necessary for cellular energy production and overall vitality.
- **Zinc**: Supports immune function, wound healing, and cell division, contributing to overall immune health and vitality.

Each of these micronutrients plays a critical role in maintaining kidney health and overall well-being, underscoring the importance of a balanced diet rich in nutrient-dense foods.

3. Sources and Recommended Intake

Obtaining adequate vitamins and minerals through diet is essential for supporting kidney health. Here are sources and recommended intake levels for key vitamins and minerals:

- **Vitamin D**: Found in fatty fish (e.g., salmon, mackerel), fortified dairy products (e.g., milk, yogurt), and sunlight exposure. Recommended intake varies, often supplemented in individuals with kidney disease.
- **Vitamin B Complex**: Found in whole grains, lean meats, dairy products, leafy greens, and fortified cereals.

Recommended daily intake varies by specific B vitamin and individual needs.

- **Vitamin C**: Found in citrus fruits (e.g., oranges, grapefruits), strawberries, kiwi, tomatoes, and bell peppers. Recommended intake is typically 75-90 mg per day for adults.
- **Folate**: Found in leafy green vegetables (e.g., spinach, kale), legumes (e.g., beans, lentils), fortified cereals, and citrus fruits. Recommended intake is 400-600 mcg per day for adults.
- **Calcium**: Sources include dairy products (e.g., milk, cheese), fortified plant-based milk alternatives (e.g., almond milk), leafy greens (e.g., collard greens, broccoli), and canned fish with bones (e.g., sardines). Recommended intake varies by age, sex, and life stage.
- **Magnesium**: Found in nuts (e.g., almonds, cashews), seeds (e.g., pumpkin seeds, sunflower seeds), whole grains (e.g., brown rice, quinoa), legumes (e.g., black beans, chickpeas), and dark chocolate. Recommended intake is around 310-420 mg per day for adults.
- **Iron**: Sources include lean meats (e.g., beef, poultry), seafood (e.g., oysters, shrimp), beans and lentils, fortified cereals, and dark leafy greens (e.g., spinach, kale). Recommended intake varies by age, sex, and life stage.
- **Zinc**: Found in meat (e.g., beef, pork), shellfish (e.g., crab, shrimp), dairy products (e.g., cheese, milk), whole grains (e.g., wheat germ, oatmeal), and legumes (e.g., chickpeas, lentils). Recommended intake is around 8-11 mg per day for adults.

It's essential to tailor intake levels based on individual health needs, kidney function, and any specific dietary restrictions or recommendations provided by healthcare providers. By incorporating a variety of nutrient-dense foods into your diet and ensuring adequate intake of essential vitamins and minerals, you can support kidney health and overall well-being. Consulting with a registered dietitian or healthcare provider can help personalize your nutrient intake to best meet your individual needs and optimize kidney function.

SPECIAL DIETARY CONSIDERATIONS

Special dietary considerations are essential for individuals managing kidney health, particularly those with chronic kidney disease (CKD) and kidney stones. This chapter explores tailored dietary plans, adjustments based on CKD stages, and specific dietary implications for managing kidney stones.

1. For Individuals with CKD

Chronic kidney disease (CKD) requires special dietary considerations to manage symptoms, slow progression, and maintain overall health:

- **Monitoring Nutrient Intake**: Individuals with CKD may need to limit certain nutrients like protein, sodium, potassium, and phosphorus to reduce stress on the kidneys and manage associated complications.
- **Balanced Diet**: Emphasize a balanced diet rich in nutrient-dense foods while controlling portions and limiting processed foods high in sodium, phosphorus, and potassium.
- **Fluid Management**: Fluid intake may need adjustment based on kidney function and fluid retention. Monitoring fluid intake helps prevent complications like edema and high blood pressure.

2. Tailored Dietary Plans

Tailored dietary plans for CKD focus on managing symptoms, slowing disease progression, and supporting overall health:

- **Protein Restriction**: Depending on CKD stage, protein intake may need to be reduced to lessen the kidneys' workload and minimize waste buildup.
- **Sodium Control**: Limiting sodium helps manage blood pressure and fluid retention, reducing strain on the kidneys.
- **Phosphorus Management**: Controlling phosphorus intake helps prevent bone and cardiovascular complications associated with CKD.

- **Potassium Balance**: Adjusting potassium intake helps manage electrolyte balance and reduce the risk of heart rhythm abnormalities.

3. Adjusting Nutrient Intake Based on CKD Stages

Nutrient requirements change as CKD progresses through stages:

- **Early Stages (Stages 1-2)**: Focus on maintaining overall health and managing risk factors such as hypertension and diabetes. Dietary adjustments may include monitoring protein and sodium intake.
- **Moderate Stages (Stages 3-4)**: More significant dietary adjustments may be necessary, including stricter limits on protein, sodium, potassium, and phosphorus to manage symptoms and slow disease progression.
- **Advanced Stage (Stage 5, End-Stage Renal Disease)**: Dialysis and/or kidney transplant may be necessary. Dietary recommendations are critical to managing complications and supporting overall health alongside medical interventions.

4. For Individuals with Kidney Stones

Kidney stones require specific dietary considerations to prevent recurrence and manage symptoms:

- **Types of Kidney Stones**: Calcium oxalate, uric acid, and other types of stones have different dietary implications.
- **Dietary Implications**:
  - **Calcium Oxalate Stones**: Limit oxalate-rich foods (e.g., spinach, rhubarb, nuts) and maintain adequate calcium intake to bind oxalate in the digestive tract.
  - **Uric Acid Stones**: Reduce purine-rich foods (e.g., organ meats, shellfish) and maintain hydration to prevent uric acid crystallization.
  - **Other Stones**: Dietary adjustments vary based on stone composition and individual factors, such as fluid intake and specific medical conditions.

5. Tailoring Your Diet

Tailoring your diet to manage kidney health involves personalized adjustments based on individual health needs, CKD stage, and kidney stone type. Consulting with a registered dietitian or healthcare provider is crucial to developing a customized nutrition plan that supports kidney function and overall well-being effectively. By following tailored dietary recommendations, individuals can optimize their nutritional intake, manage symptoms, and enhance their quality of life while maintaining kidney health.

Meal Planning and Preparation

Meal planning and preparation are essential components of maintaining kidney health, ensuring adherence to dietary guidelines, and supporting overall well-being. This chapter offers practical advice on creating kidney-friendly meal plans, daily and weekly planning tips, portion control, balanced meals, shopping strategies for kidney health, reading food labels, and effective tips for grocery shopping.

1. Creating a Kidney-Friendly Meal Plan

A kidney-friendly meal plan focuses on nutrient balance while managing intake of protein, sodium, potassium, and phosphorus:

- **Balanced Nutrients**: Incorporate a variety of foods rich in essential nutrients such as fruits, vegetables, whole grains, lean proteins, and healthy fats.
- **Individualized Approach**: Tailor meal plans to specific dietary needs and restrictions based on kidney function and health status.
- **Dietary Guidelines**: Follow recommendations from healthcare providers or registered dietitians to ensure nutritional adequacy and support kidney health.

2. Daily and Weekly Planning Tips

Effective planning ensures consistency and adherence to dietary goals:

- **Meal Prep Schedule**: Allocate time weekly to plan and prepare meals in advance, ensuring a steady supply of kidney-friendly options.
- **Batch Cooking**: Prepare large portions of meals and freeze them in individual servings for convenience and portion control throughout the week.
- **Variety and Rotation**: Plan diverse meals to maintain interest and ensure nutritional variety over time.

3. Portion Control and Balanced Meals

Maintaining proper portion sizes is crucial for managing nutrient intake:

- **Protein**: Measure portions of protein to meet daily requirements while avoiding excess that may strain kidney function.
- **Vegetables and Fruits**: Fill half of the plate with non-starchy vegetables and include fruits as part of balanced meals to add fiber and essential nutrients.
- **Whole Grains**: Choose whole grains like brown rice, quinoa, or whole wheat pasta for sustained energy and dietary fiber.

4. Shopping for Kidney Health

Strategic shopping supports a kidney-friendly diet:

- **Grocery List Preparation**: Plan meals and snacks ahead of time and create a shopping list based on kidney-friendly foods.
- **Fresh Produce**: Select fresh fruits and vegetables low in potassium and phosphorus, such as apples, berries, bell peppers, and cabbage.
- **Lean Proteins**: Choose lean cuts of meat, poultry, or fish, or opt for plant-based proteins like beans and legumes.

5. Reading Food Labels

Understanding food labels aids in making informed choices:

- **Sodium Awareness**: Check sodium levels per serving and select products with lower sodium content or opt for sodium-free alternatives.

- **Phosphorus and Potassium**: Identify phosphorus and potassium additives in processed foods and choose options lower in these minerals.
- **Ingredient Awareness**: Be mindful of hidden sources of additives, preservatives, and artificial flavors that may impact kidney health.

6. Tips for Grocery Shopping

Navigate the grocery store with kidney health in mind:

- **Perimeter Shopping**: Prioritize fresh produce, lean proteins, and dairy products typically found around the store's perimeter.
- **Minimize Processed Foods**: Limit purchases of processed foods high in sodium, phosphorus additives, and added sugars.
- **Comparative Shopping**: Compare nutrition labels to make informed choices that align with kidney-friendly dietary goals.

By incorporating these meal planning and preparation strategies, individuals can effectively manage their kidney health, adhere to dietary recommendations, and enjoy a variety of flavorful and nutritious meals. Consulting with a registered dietitian can provide personalized guidance to optimize meal plans based on individual health needs and preferences.

Recipes for Kidney Health

A well-planned diet can greatly contribute to maintaining kidney health. This chapter provides a variety of kidney-friendly recipes for breakfast, lunch, dinner, snacks, and beverages. These recipes are designed to be balanced, nutritious, and supportive of overall well-being.

Breakfast Recipes

Starting your day with a nutritious breakfast is crucial for sustained energy and kidney health.

1. Oatmeal with Berries and Flaxseeds

- **Ingredients**:
    1. 1/2 cup rolled oats
    2. 1 cup water or low-sodium almond milk
    3. 1/4 cup fresh berries (e.g., blueberries, strawberries)
    4. 1 tablespoon flaxseeds
    5. Honey or maple syrup (optional)
- **Instructions**:
    1. Cook oats in water or almond milk according to package instructions.
    2. Top with fresh berries and flaxseeds.
    3. Sweeten with a small amount of honey or maple syrup if desired.

2. Vegetable Egg White Omelet

- **Ingredients**:
    1. 3 egg whites
    2. 1/4 cup chopped bell peppers
    3. 1/4 cup chopped spinach
    4. 1/4 cup diced tomatoes
    5. 1/4 cup chopped onions
    6. 1 tablespoon olive oil
    7. Salt and pepper to taste
- **Instructions**:
    1. Heat olive oil in a non-stick skillet over medium heat.
    2. Sauté vegetables until tender.
    3. Add egg whites and cook until set.
    4. Season with salt and pepper to taste.

3. Smoothie Bowl

- **Ingredients**:
    1. 1/2 cup frozen berries
    2. 1/2 banana
    3. 1/2 cup low-sodium almond milk
    4. 1 tablespoon chia seeds
    5. 1/4 cup granola (low-sugar, kidney-friendly)
- **Instructions**:

1. Blend frozen berries, banana, and almond milk until smooth.
2. Pour into a bowl and top with chia seeds and granola.

Kidney-Friendly Options

Choose options that support kidney health and provide balanced nutrition.

1. Greek Yogurt with Fruit and Honey

- **Ingredients**:
    1. 1 cup plain Greek yogurt
    2. 1/4 cup fresh berries
    3. 1 teaspoon honey
- **Instructions**:
    1. Top Greek yogurt with fresh berries.
    2. Drizzle with honey.

2. Avocado Toast

- **Ingredients**:
    1. 1 slice whole-grain bread
    2. 1/2 avocado
    3. Lemon juice
    4. Salt and pepper to taste
- **Instructions**:
    1. Toast the bread.
    2. Mash avocado and spread it on the toast.
    3. Sprinkle with lemon juice, salt, and pepper.

Lunch and Dinner Recipes

Prepare balanced and nutritious meals for lunch and dinner that cater to kidney health.

1. Grilled Chicken Salad

- **Ingredients**:
    1. 4 oz grilled chicken breast
    2. Mixed greens
    3. 1/4 cup cherry tomatoes
    4. 1/4 cup cucumber slices

5. 1/4 cup shredded carrots
6. 1 tablespoon olive oil
7. 1 tablespoon balsamic vinegar

- **Instructions**:
    1. Slice grilled chicken breast.
    2. In a large bowl, combine mixed greens, cherry tomatoes, cucumber slices, and shredded carrots.
    3. Top with grilled chicken.
    4. Drizzle with olive oil and balsamic vinegar.

2. Baked Salmon with Asparagus

- **Ingredients**:
    1. 4 oz salmon fillet
    2. 1/2 bunch asparagus
    3. 1 tablespoon olive oil
    4. Lemon wedges
    5. Salt and pepper to taste
- **Instructions**:
    1. Preheat oven to 375°F (190°C).
    2. Place salmon and asparagus on a baking sheet.
    3. Drizzle with olive oil and season with salt and pepper.
    4. Bake for 15-20 minutes or until salmon is cooked through.
    5. Serve with lemon wedges.

3. Quinoa and Vegetable Stir-Fry

- **Ingredients**:
    1. 1 cup cooked quinoa
    2. 1/4 cup chopped bell peppers
    3. 1/4 cup chopped broccoli
    4. 1/4 cup chopped carrots
    5. 1/4 cup sliced mushrooms
    6. 1 tablespoon soy sauce (low-sodium)
    7. 1 tablespoon olive oil
- **Instructions**:
    1. Heat olive oil in a large skillet over medium heat.
    2. Add vegetables and sauté until tender.
    3. Stir in cooked quinoa and soy sauce.
    4. Cook for an additional 2-3 minutes.

Balanced and Nutritious Meals

Ensure meals are well-rounded and support kidney health.

1. Turkey and Vegetable Wrap

- **Ingredients**:
    1. 1 whole-grain tortilla
    2. 3 oz sliced turkey breast
    3. 1/4 cup shredded lettuce
    4. 1/4 cup diced tomatoes
    5. 1 tablespoon hummus
- **Instructions**:
    1. Spread hummus on the tortilla.
    2. Layer with sliced turkey, shredded lettuce, and diced tomatoes.
    3. Roll up the tortilla and slice in half.

2. Lentil Soup

- **Ingredients**:
    1. 1 cup dried lentils
    2. 4 cups low-sodium vegetable broth
    3. 1/2 cup chopped carrots
    4. 1/2 cup chopped celery
    5. 1/2 cup chopped onions
    6. 1 tablespoon olive oil
    7. Salt and pepper to taste
- **Instructions**:
    1. Heat olive oil in a large pot over medium heat.
    2. Add carrots, celery, and onions, and sauté until tender.
    3. Add lentils and vegetable broth.
    4. Bring to a boil, then reduce heat and simmer for 25-30 minutes.
    5. Season with salt and pepper to taste.

Snacks and Beverages

Incorporate healthy snack ideas and hydrating drink options to support kidney health.

1. Healthy Snack Ideas

- **Apple Slices with Almond Butter**

- o   Slice an apple and serve with 1 tablespoon almond butter.
- **Carrot and Cucumber Sticks with Hummus**
  - o   Cut carrots and cucumbers into sticks and serve with 2 tablespoons hummus.
- **Trail Mix**
  - o   Combine unsalted nuts, seeds, and dried cranberries for a kidney-friendly trail mix.

Hydrating Drink Options

Proper hydration is crucial for kidney health.

1. Infused Water

- **Ingredients**:
  1. Water
  2. Slices of lemon, cucumber, or berries
- **Instructions**:
  1. Add slices of lemon, cucumber, or berries to a pitcher of water.
  2. Let it sit in the refrigerator for a few hours before serving.

2. Herbal Tea

- **Ingredients**:
  1. Herbal tea bags (e.g., chamomile, peppermint)
  2. Water
- **Instructions**:
  1. Boil water and pour it over the herbal tea bag.
  2. Steep for 5-7 minutes and enjoy.

3. Coconut Water

- **Ingredients**:
  1. Unsweetened coconut water
- **Instructions**:
  1. Chill unsweetened coconut water in the refrigerator.
  2. Serve cold.

By incorporating these meal planning and preparation strategies, individuals can effectively manage their kidney health, adhere to dietary recommendations, and enjoy a variety of flavorful and nutritious meals. Consulting with a registered dietitian can provide personalized guidance to optimize meal plans based on individual health needs and preferences.

Eating Out and Social Situations

Maintaining a kidney-friendly diet while eating out or attending social gatherings can be challenging. However, with a bit of preparation and knowledge, you can make healthy choices that support your kidney health without feeling deprived. This chapter will provide strategies for navigating restaurant menus, making kidney-friendly choices, handling social gatherings, and staying on track during events and holidays.

Navigating Restaurant Menus

Eating out doesn't have to disrupt your kidney-friendly diet. Here are some tips to help you navigate restaurant menus and make smart choices:

1. **Research Beforehand**:
   o Check the restaurant's menu online before you go. Many restaurants provide nutritional information which can help you plan your meal.
   o Look for dishes that are grilled, baked, or steamed rather than fried or sautéed.
2. **Ask Questions**:
   o Don't hesitate to ask your server about how dishes are prepared.
   o Ask about ingredients and request modifications to better suit your dietary needs.
3. **Customize Your Order**:
   o Request sauces and dressings on the side to control the amount you consume.
   o Substitute high-sodium sides with steamed vegetables or a side salad.
   o Avoid dishes with hidden sources of sodium like soups, sauces, and processed meats.
4. **Watch Portion Sizes**:
   o Restaurant portions are often large. Consider sharing a meal, ordering a half portion, or taking leftovers home.
   o Start with a small portion and eat slowly to better gauge your hunger.

Making Kidney-Friendly Choices

When selecting dishes, focus on kidney-friendly choices to support your health:

1. **Lean Proteins**:
   - o Choose grilled chicken, fish, turkey, or lean cuts of beef.
   - o Consider plant-based proteins like beans and lentils if they fit your dietary plan.
2. **Low-Sodium Options**:
   - o Opt for dishes labeled as low sodium or ask for no added salt.
   - o Avoid cured meats, pickles, and salty snacks.
3. **Managing Potassium and Phosphorus**:
   - o Select vegetables low in potassium, such as green beans, carrots, and cauliflower.
   - o Limit high-phosphorus foods like dairy products, nuts, seeds, and certain whole grains.
4. **Healthy Sides**:
   - o Choose sides like steamed vegetables, fresh salads with low-sodium dressing, or a piece of fresh fruit.
   - o Avoid sides like fries, chips, or anything breaded and fried.

Tips for Social Gatherings

Social gatherings can pose challenges, but with some planning, you can stay on track:

1. **Eat Before You Go**:
   - o Have a small, kidney-friendly meal or snack before attending a gathering to avoid overeating.
2. **Bring a Dish**:
   - o Offer to bring a kidney-friendly dish to share. This ensures there will be something you can eat and introduces others to your dietary choices.
3. **Stay Hydrated**:
   - o Drink plenty of water throughout the event to stay hydrated and help manage your appetite.
   - o Avoid high-sodium beverages such as certain sodas and cocktails.
4. **Control Portions**:

o Take small portions of foods that may not be kidney-friendly to satisfy your cravings without overindulging.

o Fill your plate with kidney-friendly options first and add small amounts of other foods.

Staying on Track During Events and Holidays

Holidays and special events often feature indulgent foods. Here's how to stay on track:

1. **Plan Ahead**:
   o Anticipate the types of foods that will be available and plan your meals accordingly.
   o Eat lighter meals earlier in the day if you know you'll be indulging later.
2. **Healthy Alternatives**:
   o Prepare kidney-friendly versions of traditional dishes using low-sodium broths, fresh herbs, and spices.
   o Opt for baking, grilling, or steaming rather than frying.
3. **Mindful Eating**:
   o Pay attention to your hunger and fullness cues. Eat slowly, savor your food, and stop when you're satisfied.
   o Use smaller plates to help control portion sizes.
4. **Stay Active**:
   o Incorporate physical activity into your holiday routine. A walk after a meal can help with digestion and keep you active.

By implementing these strategies, you can enjoy dining out and social gatherings while maintaining a kidney-friendly diet. Remember that moderation is key, and occasional indulgences are fine as long as they fit into your overall dietary plan. Consulting with a registered dietitian can provide additional personalized guidance and support.

Supplements and Alternative Therapies

When it comes to maintaining kidney health, a balanced diet is essential, but sometimes supplements and alternative therapies can play a supportive role. This chapter explores when supplements are needed, safe supplementation practices, and the potential benefits and risks of herbal and alternative therapies.

When Supplements Are Needed

While a well-balanced diet typically provides all the necessary nutrients, certain conditions or dietary restrictions might necessitate the use of supplements:

1. **Nutrient Deficiencies**:
    o If blood tests reveal deficiencies in essential nutrients such as vitamin D, calcium, or iron, supplements may be required to correct these deficiencies.
2. **Chronic Kidney Disease (CKD)**:
    o Individuals with CKD often have specific dietary restrictions that can lead to nutrient deficiencies. For instance, the need to limit potassium and phosphorus might reduce the intake of certain fruits, vegetables, and whole grains.
3. **Post-Surgery or Illness**:
    o Recovery from surgeries, particularly kidney-related ones, or illnesses might require temporary supplementation to support healing and overall health.
4. **Dietary Restrictions**:
    o Vegetarians, vegans, or those with food allergies might need supplements to ensure they receive adequate nutrition.

Safe Supplementation for Kidney Health

When considering supplements, it is crucial to choose safe and appropriate options, especially for individuals with kidney issues:

1. **Consult a Healthcare Provider**:
    o Always consult with a healthcare provider before starting any supplement. They can provide

personalized recommendations based on your health status and needs.

2. **Avoid High-Dose Supplements**:
   o High doses of certain vitamins and minerals can be harmful. For example, excessive vitamin C can increase the risk of kidney stones, and too much vitamin A can lead to toxicity.
3. **Choose Kidney-Safe Supplements**:
   o Opt for supplements specifically formulated for kidney health, avoiding those high in potassium, phosphorus, or sodium.
4. **Monitor Levels Regularly**:
   o Regular blood tests can help monitor nutrient levels and adjust supplement dosages as needed.

Herbal and Alternative Therapies

Herbal and alternative therapies can complement traditional treatments, but it's important to be aware of their benefits and risks:

1. **Potential Benefits**:
   o Some herbal remedies and alternative therapies may offer benefits such as reducing inflammation, improving kidney function, and supporting overall health.
2. **Common Herbs and Therapies**:
   o **Cranberry**: Often used to prevent urinary tract infections, which can affect kidney health.
   o **Turmeric**: Known for its anti-inflammatory properties, it may help reduce inflammation in the kidneys.
   o **Dandelion Root**: Traditionally used as a diuretic to help the kidneys flush out excess fluid and toxins.
3. **Potential Risks**:
   o **Interactions with Medications**: Herbal supplements can interact with prescribed medications, potentially reducing their effectiveness or causing harmful side effects.
   o **Toxicity**: Some herbs can be toxic to the kidneys. For example, high doses of herbs like Aristolochia can cause severe kidney damage.
   o **Lack of Regulation**: Unlike prescription medications, herbal supplements are not strictly regulated, which can lead to variability in strength and purity.

Safe Use of Herbal Supplements

To safely incorporate herbal and alternative therapies:

1. **Consult with Healthcare Providers**:
   - o Always discuss any herbal supplements or alternative therapies with your healthcare provider to ensure they are safe and appropriate for your condition.
2. **Choose Reputable Brands**:
   - o Select products from reputable brands that follow good manufacturing practices and provide clear information about ingredients and dosages.
3. **Start with Low Doses**:
   - o Begin with the lowest effective dose to minimize the risk of side effects and monitor your body's response.
4. **Monitor Your Health**:
   - o Regularly check in with your healthcare provider to monitor how the herbal supplements are affecting your kidney function and overall health.

By understanding when supplements are needed and how to safely incorporate them into your routine, along with being cautious about herbal and alternative therapies, you can support your kidney health effectively. Always prioritize communication with your healthcare team to ensure that any supplements or therapies align with your overall treatment plan and health goals.

Monitoring and Adjusting Your Diet

Maintaining a kidney-friendly diet requires ongoing attention and adjustments. Regularly monitoring your nutritional intake and working with healthcare providers are crucial steps in ensuring your diet continues to support your kidney health. This chapter will guide you through tracking your nutritional intake, utilizing tools and apps, conducting regular check-ups, and collaborating with healthcare providers to make necessary dietary adjustments.

Tracking Your Nutritional Intake

Keeping a detailed record of what you eat helps you understand your dietary patterns and ensures you meet your nutritional needs while avoiding foods that may harm your kidneys:

1. **Daily Food Diary**:
     - Record everything you eat and drink each day. Include portion sizes, ingredients, and preparation methods.
     - Note any symptoms or reactions to specific foods to identify potential dietary triggers.
2. **Nutrient Tracking**:
     - Focus on key nutrients relevant to kidney health, such as protein, sodium, potassium, phosphorus, and fluids.
     - Use charts or spreadsheets to monitor your intake of these nutrients and ensure you stay within recommended limits.
3. **Calorie Count**:
     - Tracking your calorie intake helps manage weight, which is important for overall health and kidney function.

Tools and Apps for Monitoring Diet

Numerous tools and apps can simplify the process of tracking your diet and ensure you stay on top of your nutritional goals:

1. **Mobile Apps**:

- o **MyFitnessPal**: This app allows you to log meals, scan barcodes for nutritional information, and track key nutrients.
- o **Cronometer**: Known for its comprehensive nutrient tracking, Cronometer can help you monitor your intake of vitamins, minerals, and other dietary components.
- o **Lose It!**: This app focuses on calorie counting and includes a large database of foods to help you track your meals accurately.

2. **Wearable Devices**:
   - o Devices like Fitbit or Apple Watch can help monitor your activity levels and overall health, complementing your dietary tracking.
3. **Online Resources**:
   - o Websites like NutritionData or the USDA Food Composition Database provide detailed nutritional information about various foods, aiding in accurate tracking.
4. **Food Journals**:
   - o Traditional pen-and-paper food journals can be just as effective. They are particularly useful for those who prefer a tangible record.

Regular Check-ups and Adjustments

Regular health check-ups are essential for monitoring kidney function and making necessary dietary adjustments:

1. **Scheduled Lab Tests**:
   - o Regular blood and urine tests help monitor kidney function and detect any changes in your nutritional status.
   - o Key markers include serum creatinine, blood urea nitrogen (BUN), potassium, phosphorus, calcium, and glucose levels.
2. **Routine Doctor Visits**:
   - o Regular visits to your healthcare provider allow for ongoing assessment of your kidney health and dietary needs.
   - o Discuss any changes in your health, symptoms, or dietary challenges you face.
3. **Dietary Adjustments**:

o Based on lab results and health assessments, your healthcare provider may recommend dietary adjustments to better manage your kidney health.
o Changes may involve modifying nutrient intake, incorporating new foods, or eliminating foods that may negatively impact your kidneys.

Working with Healthcare Providers to Adjust Diet

Collaboration with healthcare providers ensures your dietary plan is both effective and safe:

1. **Registered Dietitian**:
   o Working with a registered dietitian who specializes in kidney health can provide personalized dietary guidance and meal planning.
   o A dietitian can help tailor your diet to meet your specific health needs and preferences.
2. **Nephrologist**:
   o Your nephrologist plays a crucial role in managing your kidney health and can provide insights into how your diet impacts your kidneys.
   o They can recommend tests, treatments, and dietary adjustments based on your overall health and kidney function.
3. **Regular Communication**:
   o Maintain open communication with your healthcare team. Share your food diaries, discuss challenges, and seek advice on dietary changes.
   o Regularly update them on any new symptoms or health changes to ensure your dietary plan remains appropriate.
4. **Support Groups**:
   o Consider joining support groups for individuals with kidney conditions. These groups can provide emotional support and practical advice from others who share similar experiences.

By diligently tracking your nutritional intake, utilizing available tools and apps, conducting regular check-ups, and collaborating with healthcare providers, you can effectively manage and adjust your diet to support your kidney health. This proactive approach ensures that your dietary plan remains aligned with your health goals and adapts to any changes in your condition.

Psychological and Emotional Support

Maintaining a kidney-friendly diet can be challenging not only physically but also psychologically and emotionally. Adjusting to new dietary restrictions, staying motivated, and finding support are essential for long-term success. This chapter focuses on coping with dietary changes, strategies for maintaining motivation, and identifying support systems and resources.

Coping with Dietary Changes

Adapting to a new diet can be overwhelming. Here are some strategies to help you cope with these changes:

1. **Acknowledge Your Feelings**:
   - It's natural to feel frustrated, anxious, or even sad about dietary restrictions. Acknowledge these feelings as a normal part of the adjustment process.
2. **Educate Yourself**:
   - Understanding why certain foods are restricted and how they affect your kidney health can help you make informed choices and feel more in control.
3. **Set Realistic Goals**:
   - Start with small, achievable dietary changes. Gradually incorporate more adjustments as you become more comfortable with the new diet.
4. **Create a Positive Environment**:
   - Surround yourself with supportive family and friends who understand your dietary needs and can help you stay on track.
5. **Seek Professional Guidance**:
   - A registered dietitian can provide personalized advice and meal planning, making the transition smoother and more manageable.

Strategies for Maintaining Motivation

Staying motivated to follow a kidney-friendly diet is crucial for long-term adherence. Here are some strategies to keep you on track:

1. **Set Clear Goals**:

- o Establish specific, measurable, and achievable goals related to your diet. Celebrate small victories to stay motivated.
2. **Track Your Progress**:
   - o Use a food journal or app to track your meals and monitor your progress. Seeing your improvements can boost motivation.
3. **Find Enjoyable Alternatives**:
   - o Experiment with kidney-friendly recipes and discover new foods that you enjoy. Variety and enjoyment can make dietary adherence easier.
4. **Stay Informed**:
   - o Keep up with the latest information on kidney health and nutrition. Knowledge can empower you to make better choices.
5. **Visualize Success**:
   - o Visualize the positive outcomes of maintaining a kidney-friendly diet, such as improved health and well-being. This mental imagery can strengthen your commitment.

Support Systems and Resources

Having a strong support system is vital for coping with dietary changes and maintaining motivation. Here's how to build and utilize support systems:

1. **Family and Friends**:
   - o Involve your loved ones in your dietary journey. Educate them about your needs so they can offer support and encouragement.
2. **Healthcare Team**:
   - o Regularly communicate with your healthcare providers, including your nephrologist and dietitian. They can provide guidance, answer questions, and adjust your diet as needed.
3. **Support Groups**:
   - o Join support groups for individuals with kidney conditions. Sharing experiences and advice with others who understand your challenges can be incredibly helpful.
4. **Online Communities**:

- o   Participate in online forums and social media groups focused on kidney health. These platforms can provide a wealth of information and support from people worldwide.
5. **Educational Resources**:
   - o   Utilize books, websites, and newsletters dedicated to kidney health and nutrition. Continuous learning can reinforce your dietary habits and introduce new strategies.

Finding Support Groups and Resources

Connecting with others who share similar experiences can provide emotional support and practical advice. Here are ways to find support groups and resources:

1. **Local Hospitals and Clinics**:
   - o   Many hospitals and clinics offer support groups for patients with kidney disease. Ask your healthcare provider about local options.
2. **National Kidney Foundation (NKF)**:
   - o   The NKF offers a variety of resources, including support groups, educational materials, and events for individuals with kidney disease.
3. **American Association of Kidney Patients (AAKP)**:
   - o   The AAKP provides resources, advocacy, and support groups for kidney patients and their families.
4. **Online Platforms**:
   - o   Websites like Facebook and Reddit host numerous groups focused on kidney health. Search for groups that match your interests and needs.
5. **Community Centers**:
   - o   Check with local community centers or libraries for information on support groups and educational workshops.

By embracing psychological and emotional support, you can better manage the challenges of maintaining a kidney-friendly diet. Coping with dietary changes, staying motivated, and utilizing support systems and resources are crucial steps in ensuring your diet supports your kidney health and overall well-being.

Conclusion

As we conclude "Nutritional Guidelines for Maintaining Kidney Health," let's revisit the essential points we've covered and underscore the importance of nutrition in maintaining optimal kidney health. This chapter will offer final thoughts and encouragement to help you stay proactive in managing your kidney health through a well-balanced diet.

Recap of Key Points

1. **Understanding the Kidneys**:
   - The kidneys are vital organs responsible for filtering waste, balancing electrolytes, and maintaining fluid balance.
   - Common kidney diseases such as chronic kidney disease (CKD) and kidney stones can significantly impact kidney function and overall health.
2. **Basics of Kidney-Friendly Nutrition**:
   - Essential nutrients for kidney health include protein, potassium, phosphorus, sodium, and fluids.
   - Balancing these nutrients and maintaining proper hydration are crucial for supporting kidney function.
3. **The Role of Protein**:
   - Protein needs vary based on individual health conditions, with a focus on moderate intake for those with CKD.
   - Sources of kidney-friendly proteins include both plant-based and animal-based options, with an emphasis on portion control.
4. **Managing Potassium and Phosphorus Intake**:
   - Potassium and phosphorus play critical roles in the body, but their levels must be managed carefully to prevent complications in kidney patients.
   - A balanced intake of these minerals helps maintain proper bodily functions and avoid issues like hyperkalemia and hyperphosphatemia.
5. **Sodium and Fluid Management**:
   - Excessive sodium intake can lead to high blood pressure and fluid retention, exacerbating kidney problems.
   - Proper hydration is essential, but fluid intake should be balanced to avoid overburdening the kidneys.

6. **Vitamins and Minerals**:
   - o Essential micronutrients support overall health and kidney function.
   - o Specific vitamins and minerals, such as vitamin D and calcium, require careful management in individuals with kidney issues.
7. **Special Dietary Considerations**:
   - o Tailored dietary plans for individuals with CKD and kidney stones can help manage these conditions and prevent further complications.
   - o Adjusting nutrient intake based on disease stages and types of kidney stones is critical.
8. **Meal Planning and Preparation**:
   - o Creating a kidney-friendly meal plan involves daily and weekly planning, portion control, and balanced meals.
   - o Shopping tips and reading food labels are essential for making informed dietary choices.
9. **Recipes for Kidney Health**:
   - o Incorporating kidney-friendly recipes for breakfast, lunch, dinner, snacks, and beverages can make dietary adherence enjoyable and sustainable.
10. **Eating Out and Social Situations**:
    - o Navigating restaurant menus and making kidney-friendly choices in social gatherings helps maintain dietary goals.
    - o Staying on track during events and holidays is possible with proper planning and awareness.
11. **Supplements and Alternative Therapies**:
    - o Understanding when supplements are needed and how to use them safely is crucial for kidney health.
    - o Herbal and alternative therapies may offer benefits but should be approached with caution.
12. **Monitoring and Adjusting Your Diet**:
    - o Tracking nutritional intake, using tools and apps, and conducting regular check-ups help in maintaining a kidney-friendly diet.
    - o Working with healthcare providers ensures that dietary adjustments are made as needed.
13. **Psychological and Emotional Support**:
    - o Coping with dietary changes and maintaining motivation are essential for long-term adherence.

o   Support systems, including family, friends, and healthcare providers, play a significant role in emotional well-being.

Importance of Nutrition in Maintaining Kidney Health

Nutrition is a cornerstone of kidney health. A well-balanced diet tailored to your specific needs can:

- Slow the progression of kidney disease.
- Prevent complications associated with kidney conditions.
- Improve overall quality of life and well-being.

By understanding and implementing the dietary guidelines outlined in this book, you can take proactive steps to support your kidney health and manage any existing conditions effectively.

Final Thoughts and Encouragement

Embarking on a journey to maintain kidney health through diet may seem challenging at first, but remember that every small step you take makes a significant difference. Here are some final thoughts and encouragement to keep you motivated:

- **Stay Informed**: Continuously educate yourself about kidney health and nutrition. Knowledge is empowering and can help you make better choices.
- **Be Patient and Persistent**: Dietary changes take time and effort. Be patient with yourself and persistent in your efforts to maintain a kidney-friendly diet.
- **Seek Support**: Don't hesitate to reach out to healthcare providers, support groups, and loved ones. Their encouragement and guidance can make your journey easier.
- **Celebrate Progress**: Acknowledge and celebrate your successes, no matter how small. Every positive change is a step towards better kidney health.

Staying Proactive About Kidney Health Through Diet

Being proactive about your kidney health means taking charge of your diet and making informed decisions. Regularly monitor your nutritional intake, stay engaged with your healthcare team, and adjust your diet as needed. By doing so, you can enhance your kidney function, prevent complications, and lead a healthier, more fulfilling life.

Remember, you have the power to make a positive impact on your kidney health through the choices you make every day. Stay committed to your dietary goals, and you'll be well on your way to maintaining optimal kidney health.

Thank you for joining us on this journey through "Nutritional Guidelines for Maintaining Kidney Health." We hope this book has provided you with valuable insights and practical tools to support your kidney health through nutrition. Stay informed, stay motivated, and most importantly, stay healthy.

ABOUT THE AUTHOR

Sunday Ekele is a multifaceted professional renowned for his expertise as an author, health specialist, and counselor. With a passion for empowering individuals to achieve holistic wellness and personal growth, Sunday has dedicated his career to blending insights from health sciences with profound psychological counseling.

As an accomplished author, Sunday Ekele has authored numerous enlightening works that delve into mental health, personal development, and the intricate dynamics of human relationships. His writing style is known for its clarity, empathy, and practical wisdom, making complex concepts accessible to readers from all walks of life.

In the realm of health specialization, Sunday Ekele brings a wealth of knowledge and experience, having advised and guided countless individuals on their journey to physical and mental well-being. His approach integrates cutting-edge research with compassionate care, aiming not only to treat symptoms but to address underlying causes and promote sustainable health practices.

Beyond his professional achievements, Sunday Ekele is recognized for his advocacy in promoting mental health awareness and holistic living within communities. Through workshops, seminars, and public speaking engagements, he strives to educate and inspire others to prioritize self-care and emotional well-being.